CONQUERING

MOUNT TA~TA

How I conquered breast cancer
~ *without losing my sense of humor.*

By L. G. Ransom

Sentinel Press
Washington D.C. USA

ISBN-13:978-1481807494
ISBN-10:1481807498
LCCN: 2013903455

Printed in the United States of America.

Preface

Let's get one thing straight: cancer sucks. If you're reading this book, I'm pretty sure you've got a good idea what the title is all about. I'm guessing that you either have cancer yourself, you've already been through cancer, or you know someone who's been diagnosed with it. By Mount Ta-Ta, I don't mean a mountain half way across the world from the Americas; I mean breasts ~ otherwise known as boobies, knockers, the girls, the goddesses, the rack, and many other quaint and colorful acronyms.

What happens to our darling idols during breast cancer is not fun nor is it neat and clean nor is it anything to laugh at. Please don't misunderstand me; I don't mean to tread on any toes. Yes, I know there's absolutely nothing comical or funny or witty about breast cancer, but you've got to admit that some of the weird situations it exposes you to are pretty damned amusing ~ if you're brave enough to laugh at them.

Cancer is something everyone lives in fear of. It completely takes over your life and doesn't always change it for the better. But when I got that dreaded diagnosis for myself, I made the decision early on that I'd try my best not to let it rob me of my sense of humor. That God-given, quirky sense of absurdity saw me through my darkest days, and I was told over and over by other women to please pass it on.

I don't know if you'll find parts of my story humorous or not, but if it can be of help to someone else, then I'm happy to share it. I've always thought that laughter, at its core, is the very best medicine ~ in my humble opinion, anyway.

With something like breast cancer, simply getting through the process is long and arduous and takes an enormous amount of willpower. Finding the amusing side of things, for me, was the only way to keep going, and I'm convinced it's the easiest way to heal and get on with life. But enough about that ~ let me tell you about me, or, more specifically, let me tell you about my stormy climb up tumorous Mount Ta-Ta and back down again, for I really did conquer the biggest mountain of my life.

Conquering Mount Ta Ta

Acknowledgements

My entire journey through cancer would not have been possible without the loving support of my family; especially my kids Katey Sue and Nicholas, my husband David, and my parents Mike and Bonnie Green. You kept me fighting, even during the times when I didn't want to anymore.

I would especially like to thank my cancer buddy ~ my aunt, Nancy Hammett, who was diagnosed with her last round of cancer just as I was going through the trauma of my mastectomy. No matter how tired or sick she was with her own treatments, she always took the time to write me a happy note or call to remind me to eat more chocolate. It's unfathomable to me that I survived this insidious disease, and she didn't, but her glowing spirit will always live on in my heart

Conquering Mount Ta Ta

1
Facing Mount Ta-Ta

To start at the beginning, let me just say that I'm not a very large person. Don't let the fact that I'm five-foot-five fool you; it's all in the legs. I'm not model thin or anything, but I wear a size four wedding ring. And you can forget adult size watches and bracelets: the ones that fit me best come from the children's department. In fact, the only thing that could ever be called "large" about me was my chest.

I spent most of my teen years flatter than a pancake. Then, all of a sudden, I woke up in my twenties to boom-chicka-wow-wow. Mind you, I was not nearly as well-endowed as some reality-TV ladies who would completely overshadow me, but by thirty-five, after the birth of my second child, they got, in my opinion, ridiculously massive. I'm talking so substantial that the local maternity stores didn't carry anything large enough, so I had to special order my nursing bras from Canada via the Internet. They were so enormous that my poor little son was faced with the awful prospect of latching on to a melon twice the size of his head. It was a race against time for him to eat or be suffocated—and is probably the reason he can't stand to drink milk to this day.

I had been assured by every book I had read, and by the mournful sobs of several friends, that the girls were sure to disappear as soon as the babies were weaned ~ and they did…sort of. By the time my youngest was two, I had been reduced to a respectably large size DD cup, but to my pitiful dismay, instead of the nice rounded peaks of my youth, I was left with what could only be described as something resembling the flopping ears of a hound dog. Thank the good Lord for the invention of sports bras. If you wear two at once, they give great lift and prevent that annoying side-to-side flop that burns your underarms ~ if you remember to powder them on warm days.

I've always had fibrocystic disease. On my very first visit to the gynecologist, she warned me that my breasts were very lumpy and that I'd have to watch them closely as I got older. But what does that really mean to a young person anyway? They've always had lumps and bumps and ached like crazy during certain times of the month. After the kids were born, they both pointed in awkward directions if they didn't have adequate support or corset-like encouragement to do otherwise; that was just normal. So self-exams and all the "tell-tale signs" of what to look for were pretty much useless. There was always some pebble to feel in there, and after awhile, I just pretty much ignored the rocky terrain and placed my faith in that modern inquisitional device that is coquettishly named ~ the mammogram.

2
Mammogram Trail

Every good climbing expedition begins at the bottom of the mountain ~ usually with a very innocuous looking trail inviting you to delve deeper into the deep, dark woods. I've always maintained that whoever invented the mammogram was a secret sadist. I mean, seriously, let's think about this for a moment. Women dutifully line up and expose their naked breast to a little, freezing-cold plastic tray which then tries to electronically compress it flatter than a pancake in an unfeeling, mechanical vice.

"Hold your breath for a few seconds, please," the technician always says pleasantly. *Hold my breath? Oh my God, I can't even suck in enough air to hold; just get the damn picture and let it go!*

I'd been faithfully getting mammograms every year since I was about thirty years old. I called it my yearly "racking" and have always secretly felt that we really haven't progressed much from the Flagellants of old. They whipped themselves senseless to drive off the plague in medieval Europe; whereas, here we are a few hundred years later, compacting our privates to the point of tears in an attempt to eradicate cancer. Human evolution is such a fascinating thing.

In more recent times, I've heard that some insurance companies have been getting a bit prickly over the cost of a mammo every single year. There are those who argue that, if you're under a certain age or your previous ones are all clear, then you really don't need that particular exam on an annual basis. Every other year, or even every so many years, would be just fine. Honestly, just twist my rubber arm on that one. You mean you don't want me to bare all to the malevolent torture press? That's fine with me. I was going on my fifteenth anniversary with those suckers. So I skipped a year.

In the summer of 2012, however, I really couldn't rationalize my way out of getting one. I wasn't particularly worried. I knew the drill: disrobe, present boob, squeeze the life out of said boob, try to refrain from using the worst of the foul language known to me, repeat on the opposite side, thank the tech nicely with a forced smile, and then go home and wait for the inevitable phone call.

Every time, like clockwork, the phone would ring, and there would be a sweet voice assuring me that all was fine, but please come back in for an ultrasound ~ just to make sure. Been there, done that, no sweat. It's a nice, quiet free hour, with no cell phone, no housework, and no refereeing between my children. The radiologist would usually come in, tell me that I have very fibrous breasts full of liquid cysts, but there is no sign of cancer, and I'd be on my way back in traffic on the interstate with six thousand or so other parents trying to get home before school lets out. On a whim, I even happily paid the extra fifty bucks and splurged on the newest 3-D version ~ hey, my kids get to go to 3-D movies, why can't I have a 3-D mammo? *Does it come with the special glasses?*

I knew something was up this time when the radiologist announced at the prophesied ultrasound that he needed to inject my left breast with a dye contrast. *Inject? Dye? Huh?* I must have looked like a deer in the headlights because he immediately assured me that he'd numb the skin first with Novocain, and once the surface was numb, he'd inject more Novocain deeper down so that I wouldn't feel the dye injection at all.

Let's stop and think about this for a second. You, a male doctor who is not my husband, are holding my left breast casually in your gloved hand while telling me that you're getting ready to inject dye into it just below the nipple ~ with a four-inch metal needle. However, it will all be okay because you're going to give me two other injections ~ with a six-inch needle ~ first. *Are you freakin' serious?* I had some very choice words on the tip of my tongue, but for some unknown pathetic reason, all speech eluded me, and I found myself simply nodding in meek, modest, and compliant acquiescence ~ allowing the whole thing to occur in silence.

Oh, but wait ~ it gets even better. Once the dye was in and he'd taken the second set of ultrasound pictures, they had to race me back down the main hall, in my hospital gown, to the dreaded torture chamber for yet another 3-D mammogram. This time the tech very sweetly asked, as I was unceremoniously gripped in the jaws of boob death, if I could just bend my legs and contort my body around the side of the machine so she could get a better angle. In response, I maliciously bled both blood and dye contrast from my injection sites all over the tray.

From there, I waited yet again in the tiny back waiting room with other nervous, similarly white-robed women who were all waiting anxiously to hear their dreaded fate. Even at this point, I wasn't too worried. It was just one more step in the mysterious world of mammo doctors doing their "thing." I read my book, wiggled my toes in impatient frustration, and was totally unprepared for the news that came next.

"Unfortunately, what I thought I saw on the 3-D is really there, and the ultrasound and the dye contrast have confirmed it. We need to schedule you for a needle biopsy."

Huh? ~ wait a minute. This was entirely new territory, and the thin, little cotton robe I was wearing did nothing for the chill that ran down my spine. The doctor gave me a few encouraging words and then left me to the nurse, who gave me some sort of low down on what would happen next. At least, I think she did, because I really don't actually remember all that much after that. All I can accurately recall is that the nurse walked me down to a never-before-visited, back checkout counter, and a biopsy was scheduled.

Conquering Mount Ta Ta

3
Down Biopsy Slope

I'll admit it: I was nervous about the needle biopsy. I'd had biopsies before ~ on other areas ~ and they'd been pretty painful. My experience this time, however, was fairly blasé. Now, I freely admit that it might have been the Lorazapam I'd demanded that is recoloring my memories of it with shades of sunflowers and rainbows ~ that's really good stuff you know ~ but it was a very quick and simple process this time around.

Just like before, I undressed and presented myself bare chest up on the table; smugly gratified at the exclamations of the doctor and nurses over the massive purple, black, red, and yellow bruises I sported from the dye-contrast torture a few days before. There were a few pricks of Novocain, and then there were two little pops, kind of like a plastic toy gun my son would play with, for each of the five samples taken ~ ten pinches in all.

It was over so fast that my husband had barely sat down in the waiting room before the radiologist came out to tell him that we were done. In fact, so little time had passed that he was firmly convinced (and I think this totally, unfairly, and unnecessarily maligns me) that the doctor was coming out to tell him that they had to delay the procedure because I'd decompensated and was wailing hysterically on the table. *Please*! I'm a black belt in Tae Kwon Do. I only wail hysterically when they tell me there are no other women to spar with in my age group, and I get put up against some eighteen-year-old boy who should be on the varsity football team instead of in "featherweight" martial arts.

I'll be completely honest with you here: the hardest part about the biopsy was the waiting. I went in on a Thursday morning and faced the entire weekend knowing that the office was closed, and no results would be available until the following week. Nonpulsed, I returned to work at Girl Scout camp the next day and simply went on with life ~ albeit, a little gingerly. (Once the Novocain and Lorazapam wear off, even a sports bra hurts.)

Fortunately for me, it was a very busy weekend, but then again, weekends are always insanely busy at our house. I'm your classic, super ADD adult who charges through life head on ~in six directions at all times ~ and just can't sit still if I try. I'm even ADD about my OCD. I usually find a brand new obsession every three to six months.

At this particular time in my life, I was: a full-time

mom to a thirteen-year-old girl and a nine-year-old boy, a Girl Scout leader, a Cub Scout Leader, a Girl Scout Service Unit Manager, a black belt in Tae Kwon Do, an aspiring science-fiction writer, a photographer, an artist, a pre-school Sunday school teacher, and a hockey rink mom and rink wife. And then there were all my kids' other after-school activities I shuttled them to.

This particular weekend, I had just wrapped up volunteering at the last of three summer day camps, the basement was still under construction after an early-summer flood, I had the kids' school yearbook to work on, the photos from a week at vacation bible school to sort and post, my daughter's ice skating and singing lessons, and my son's travel hockey team tryouts.

I had it very firmly cemented in my mind that the biopsy would come back negative, and all the fretting and worry would be for nothing. *Yesterday can't be changed, tomorrow hasn't happened, and the present of today needs attending to.* I'd lived by that motto for years, but I had absolutely no idea how much it would be challenged.

As it turns out, my parents just happened to be visiting from overseas, and they and everyone else I encountered assured me that these things almost always turn out perfectly fine. I had tons of encouragement from friends who all agreed that this was sure to be a non-event ~ just as my other biopsies had been. (Well, except for the one that led to my hysterectomy three years before, but that's an entirely different story.) I chastised myself repeatedly ~ all weekend ~ for allowing my overly active imagination to take over and soar out of control. I focused instead on my work and my kids, and if any stray thoughts of mammograms and needles and biopsies crossed my mind, I channeled them into considering how I could weave the tale into one of the two books I was working on. That said, it came as a complete and utter shock when the phone call came very early on Monday morning.

4

Waterfalls

Early morning phone calls from the doctor ~ especially on Monday mornings ~ never seem to bear good news. That particular Monday morning was pretty crappy. I woke up to the death of one of my prettiest ten-inch fantail goldfish, Sushi, and had to quickly send him along on his golden oceanly voyage before my children woke up ~ which left little time for coffee. The van was acting up, my head hurt, and neither of my children could seem to say anything nice to one another: to the point where thermal nuclear war between them seemed inevitable. It was also a really bad hair day. I had foolishly assumed that a perm was the solution to my stubbornly stick-straight locks, but the summer's high humidity had left me looking less like Rapunzel and more like a giant poodle on steroids. Needless to say, I was a little grumpy and not necessarily in the best of moods when the phone rang.

"There's no good way to say this," my gynecologist informed me. "You have breast cancer, but you're going to be fine."

Fine? I thought to myself ~ the numb, dumbstruck feeling crawling over me like a dentist's injection of Novocain into my jaw. *I'm not gonna be fine. I have a nine-year-old. I have a thirteen-year-old. I'm not gonna be fine ever again.* All I could think about was the trauma I was about to inflict on my family. I honestly could have cared less about me in that moment: it was my children and my husband and my parents. No, I wasn't *fine* by any means, and I instinctively knew I never would be again.

You can do two things when faced with a life changing diagnosis. You can either curl up in the fetal position and wail at the injustice of it all or you can fight. For me, failure was not an option. As I mentioned earlier, I'm a proud, middle-aged female black belt in martial arts, and that moment, for me, became the moment I mentally donned my sparring gear, entered the ring, and focused my mind on the total destruction of my opponent. As I numbly took down the names of the all the doctors I was now about to come under the care of, I breathed heavily, found my center, and called up that force from the gut that allows you to focus for sparring. "*I don't have cancer,*" I thought to myself, "*my body has cancer. My mind is clear and can overcome this. I still have my will to fight.*"

Once I had written down all the names and phone numbers of my new cancer team, my gynecologist began a long recitation of all the options that now lay before me: from herbs and meditation all the way up to a full mastectomy and radiation with chemo. She assured me there was plenty of time to weigh my options and decide the best course for me. The only option for me, though, was the one that assured I was gonna *live*. I had two children ~ I had to.

But then I thought about my hair. Suddenly I didn't care if I looked like a poodle. I burst into tears ~ firmly proving once and for all that I'm absolutely as chicken-livered and vain as I've always dreaded I was. Misunderstanding what was really going on, my family rallied around me with hugs and kisses and support. However, true to form, once the tears had dried up, I was able to sniff loudly and say, *"Well, I guess this means I can let the Cub Scouts paint my head as a popcorn-selling reward."*

Conquering Mount Ta Ta

5
Up MRI Ridge

Whoever invented the MRI apparatus for scanning breasts should be hung by a slip knot around his testicles until a full session of scanning breast tissue is over with. That's my opinion of course, but that's just me. I know it was a man that did it because men developed stirrups for the gynecology table, the underwire bra, and I think it was a man that decided an episiotomy was better than tearing during childbirth. (*Okay, that last one is debatable; I admit it*).

By this point in my journey, I was pretty damn vulnerable. My earlier resolve to conquer this thing was swinging back and forth like the pendulum of an ancient grandfather clock. Back and forth, up and down: my emotions went everywhere. As it happened, this was the same time as the summer Olympics and the kids had just watched a little blurb on the news about the strength and perseverance of an Olympic athlete who had just lost his mother to breast cancer. My nine-year-old son had turned to me with an utterly stunned look and said, "Wait…you can *die* from breast cancer?" I had never wanted to burst into tears faster or louder than at that moment, but I didn't. I turned to him calmly and very firmly told him, "Yes, but I'm not gonna die." Then I excused myself and ate three chocolate brownies with a huge glass of red wine.

My assurances seemed to pacify my son for the time being, but, as they placed the IV in my arm for the dye contrast of the MRI, I suddenly burst into tears and promptly nearly passed out. Fainting is very embarrassing for a black belt; it's certainly not encouraged. I turned bright reddish purple in shame as they quickly lowered my head and fussed over me ~ concerned more that I was experiencing an allergic reaction to the dye test than the fact that I was just feeling humiliated over having an old fashioned, mortifying fit of vapors.

I feel so sorry for the MRI patient scheduled behind me. I was one of the first up for the day, and I know I totally blew the department's whole schedule to hell after that. Someone actually went upstairs and got my surgeon's nurse practitioner to come in to talk with me. Once she realized that I was probably just mild tempered and prone to silly female hysterics (*um…not!*), she sat me back up, and with the MRI tech on the other side, they gently walked me into the scanning room with soft, encouraging words. It was totally pathetic.

I've had MRI's before ~ but not one for breasts. When they scanned my neck after I took a kick to the throat, I'd lain on my back. When I had a stress fracture in my left kicking foot, I'd also lain on my back. Somehow, I just assumed they'd lay me on my back again, but maybe they would slide me further into the tube. I couldn't have been more wrong.

As I was led in, I couldn't help staring at the table; it was all cut up. In the bed, there were two little squares which the tech quickly pulled down into rectangles. I was then asked to lie face down on the table, with my forehead against a top pad, my face in an open square. Each boob was pushed through one of the rectangles so that they could dangle freely in the icy air toward the open floor. This is how I know the breast MRI apparatus was designed by a man. Not only was I squeezing a set of overly large round girls through an opening in the table, I was squeezing them through rectangular holes. *Please ~ only a man would design something like that; I just know it.*

I'm not sure how long the actual scan lasted, but it was pretty stifling and uncomfortable. The pad across my forehead was the only thing supporting my head and neck, and the only things I could see were through a strategically placed mirror below me. It actually gave me a little motion sickness, and try as I might, I had more than one quick, little panic attack. Just when I was positive that they had to be finished, I heard the voice of the tech announcing that they were only just ready to inject the dye contrast. *What the freckled varmint ~ seriously?*

25

Taking a deep breath, I focused on counting to ten: in Korean, then Spanish, then French, and then Hungarian. I tried German as well, but those memories have apparently been totally eradicated. Since this was about the extent of my recollection of foreign language, I then focused on figuring out the foulest possible phrase I could conjure for a dye-contrast boob MRI. Unfortunately, I don't think I can actually print out those words and still retain the mom-respect of my kids ~ although, my son might appreciate them.

After what seemed like hours, the tech's voice once again broke through the headphones that they were almost finished. Then she paused a second, and I heard, "*Oh, wow!*" before the line cut off. The "*Oh, wow*" unnerved me a bit. I mean, I had just gotten through mulling over the foulest possible language to describe their breast MRI, and I was a little panicked I might have accidentally said some of those words out loud and been recorded. However, the significance of that "*Oh, wow*" wasn't to be known for several more days.

As it turns out, the MRI could see my little, biopsied tumor very clearly, but it could also see a second tiny tumor forming just below it ~ deeper into the tissue. My left lymph had lit up with the dye contrast ~ and so had hundreds of tiny little spots in both the left and the right breasts. All the doctors assured me that the results were not nearly as bad as I was taking them (which was slightly better than a screaming two-year-old who's skinned her knees on the tarmac), but it pressed me even harder into making my decisions quickly.

6
A Split in the Road

There's really nothing humorous in this little section, but I think it needs to be included so that I'm not misunderstood later on by the choices I made in my treatment. Far be it from me to pass judgment on how other women handle their choices in regard to breast cancer. There is not one right way and not one right option. There is only the one choice that one woman can make about her one diagnosis, given all the information from her doctors and the possibilities presented her. She must, in all cases, make the choice that she believes in her heart is right for her. What follows in this little blurb are the choices made by me, and they shouldn't be used as any type of guide or advice as to what others should do.

Having grown up a doctor's daughter and having very briefly gone through a few years of medical school myself, I think I had a slightly different insight into the world of cancer outcomes of the generation before me. I wouldn't say I'm entirely in favor of more aggressive medical treatment, but I certainly wasn't opposed to getting it done right the first time.

I have a very good friend whose mother was diagnosed with breast cancer in the seventies and through herbal medicines, diet and exercise; she has found herself cancer free some forty years later. However, I also knew many of my father's patients who had gone that route and lost their battles within a few years.

Growing up, I always heard my father council, "Do both. Holistic healing, diet, exercise, and meditation are as critically important as your attitude and everything medical science has to offer." The phrase, *"Never underestimate the power of positive thought,"* ~ be it prayer, meditation, or simply good wishes ~ was a huge part of my upbringing. As a physician though, my dad also strongly believed in the power of modern technology, disease-specific medicines, and proven medical treatments. The latter became my choice.

I knew Tamoxifen would not be an option. I had estrogen-receptive, invasive, ductile breast cancer, and it responds really well to that drug. I also knew I had to have at least a partial mastectomy. The holistic side of me, however, wanted to avoid radiation and chemotherapy infusions at all costs ~ if possible. I was already on a pretty good antioxidant regime and was in pretty good shape (except for the extra ten pounds middle age gifted me and the five pounds drowning my cancer sorrows in chocolate packed on), and I had a family cancer history that was a bit dicey.

Fortunately, I had my dad for guidance, and I had the bonus of a few years of med school ~ the latter of which helped tremendously in my ability to do research and understand the terminology and pharmacology. I could, in no way, professionally read the mammogram pictures of the MRI report, but I could interpret the gist of it and talk intelligently to my doctors about it.

In the end, the conclusion was pretty clear. Although my tumor was small and caught early on, another was already growing. Breast cancer in "young" women, under 50 like myself, tends to be far more aggressive than cancers that develop later in life. The left side had slightly inflamed lymph nodes, and the dye contrast had lit up both breasts and the lymph like a Christmas tree. Although the radiologist insisted there was no evidence that so many dye hits meant more cancer was already forming, I knew enough to know that this wasn't good.

My immediate options were to: (1) do more MRI-based biopsies to see exactly what we were dealing with, (2) do a partial lumpectomy for the known tumors, as well as radiation and chemotherapy infusions (3) do a left-side mastectomy, with radiation and chemotherapy or (4) do a full mastectomy ~ which would nix the need for radiation and possibly chemotherapy infusions as well.

I am generally of the opinion that more is not always better; however, I had known too many people who had opted for the lumpectomy or partial mastectomy and then had to go back two or three years later to remove the other side when the cancer came back. Plus, I knew that, with a full mastectomy, my chances of having to go through radiation and chemo infusions were much less ~ especially with an MRI that looked like a Lite-Brite.

In the end, it came down to this: no more biopsies, no more tests. Whatever I had in other areas of the breast would not change the fact that I already knew I had cancer and needed to treat it. Besides, if you really think about it, reconstruction is reconstruction. At the very least, I already knew I was going to have to cut out at least half of my left breast. Once that was completed I'd need to do reconstruction to make it look normal. But after that was done, I would need reconstruction on the right to make it look like the left.

They were also going to give me a mammogram every six months to see if any of those glowing highlights in the right breast turned into real cancer. If cancer did strike again, then they would take the right side off this time and reconstruct it again so that it matched the left. *Does anyone else besides me think this is slightly ridiculous?*

I gave them as serious a look as I could give them and said I wanted a double mastectomy. I mean, was there really any choice? Just cut the dang hound ears off along with the cancer and give me a full set of brand new, perfectly perky boobs. In reality, I knew my choice was far more serious than that, but like I said, you've got to look on the bright side of things, or you'll never get through this.

7
Base Camp

The one bad thing about growing up a doctor's daughter is that by the time you're ready to be referred out to all the doctors your dad sent his patients to when they faced cancer, they've retired. Finding a good team is essential to your survival. They have to know each other, coordinate with each other, and be totally devoted to your success. In this day and age of modern health care, I began to wonder if that were really possible. It turns out that yes, it is, but you'd better be ready to become your own best advocate.

This was, however, completely new territory for me. For the first time in my life, I was placing my care into the hands of doctors who, with only a very few exceptions, I did not know. I was trusting them with my life and felt an enormous pressure to get it right.

Let me say, I adore my oncologist. Until recently he

played recreation league adult hockey like my husband ~ so what's not to like, eh? Besides, he was one of the few doctors that was around in my dad's time. In fact, he was my gynecologist's oncologist, he was my daughter's middle school teacher's oncologist, and he was that teacher's mother's oncologist. I had complete confidence in him from the very beginning ~ which was critical ~ but I had a harder time trying to find a brand new mastectomy surgeon and reconstruction surgeon.

In the end, I simply took a leap of faith. I went with the best recommendations of the hospital that my oncologist worked through. Now-a-days, there's a whole computer network, called a portal, which is geared to coordinate all the doctors and all their information. I needed to find a team that could coordinate with this portal and my chosen hospital, so I held my breath and made the appointments.

In reality, it turns out that this "portal" system works about as well as any virus-infected Internet system. I was constantly double booked with my appointments at the same time, at different offices, and with no hope of any symmetry or coordination. Besides, if they were supposedly sharing all this info, then why did I still have to fill out mountains of the same paperwork at every office? At one point, everything got held up, because I had signed a paper on the wrong line ~ despite the fact that I had signed it in the right place at another office.

I certainly didn't see anything high tech or efficient about it. Besides, after the first visit to my oncologist, the system never once updated any of my labs. But I guess it made them feel better to say they had it.

Fortunately, by coordinating through one program, I ended up with some of the best in the business. After the rounds of initial meet-and-greets were over, I felt comfortable with my team and ready to get on with it.

The *"young"* female surgeon who was handling the actual mastectomy was about my age and seemed the only one not overly happy with my choice of a double mastectomy ~ but she'd do it. I think she felt it was overkill, but she admitted that she could see my point about wanting to avoid radiation and chemo infusions if I could, and she also understood I didn't want to have to come back and do it all over again if the right side developed cancer. The plastic surgeon was a peach. I considered him to be much younger than any plastic surgeon/boob specialist had a right to be ~ like, practically my daughter's age for goodness sake ~ but he had the confidence of my surgeons and his opinion on the double was: *"Hey, it makes my job easier."* My oncologist, GYN, primary doctor, and my dad ~ in unison ~ agreed with my decision that a double mastectomy, given my history, was the best possible option. So with my team assembled, I took a deep breath and moved forward toward the summit. Like a woman in labor, I zeroed in on my focus object: *to be cancer free, with the brand new, perfect breasts of a twenty-year-old.*

Conquering Mount Ta Ta

8
Altitude Sickness

Once the date for my mastectomy was set, the waiting seemed to take forever. There was a delay in coordinating the two surgeons' schedules with the hospital, and then a death in the family of one of my surgeons delayed things even more. In the meantime, we decided to use the lull to take the family on vacation in Alberta, Canada, and then focus on getting both kids back to school. I filled my days staying as busy as I possibly could ~which wasn't too hard ~ and meditating in the quiet moments to quell the anxiety and focus on the positive energy I'd need to get through this. By myself, this was relatively easy, but life is never just about yourself, is it?

One thing I was totally unprepared for was the look of anguish, and the outpouring of sympathy everyone gave me when I told them the news. I just couldn't fathom why everyone, even my husband, would reach out and hug me or cry over me as if I were deathly ill. I felt fine; even the bruises from the biopsy were healing.

Perhaps it was denial, but in my mind, I wasn't just gonna lie down and let them plant flowers over me. My thirteen-year-old wailed when we told her the news. My husband, who's a big tough lawyer and hockey player, cried and hugged me over and over. My parents tried hard to mask it, but you could see the strain of worry and concern in their eyes. They hugged me over and over and promised we'd get through it. Only my nine-year-old, when he was first told mommy was "sick," looked at me and said, "So? How long 'till you're better?" *My point exactly*!

For the first few weeks, I was angrier than sin. Not, mind you, angry at the cancer ~ I was angry at the reactions of everyone who found out I had cancer. This isn't to say I didn't have my terrified moments when I cried hysterically into my pillow, but for the most part, I simply couldn't deal with everyone around me and their reactions to it. I began avoiding people like the plague.

Yes, I had cancer, but I was gonna live through it. Period. End of story. I felt so incredibly weird and uncomfortable that all my family and friends were buying pink ribbons and that my son wanted a giant pink ribbon to wear on his hockey jersey and pink tape for his stick. They were all rallying around me like I had stage-five, terminal, nothing-you-can-do-about-it cancer. I felt like there were so many other women ~ past and present ~ who deserved that kind of support and tribute more than I did. It made me uncomfortable.

I had one little tumor which had reached out and spread into another little tumor. Why would anyone wear a pink ribbon for that, when there were so many far more deserving women? When there were women who had battled so much harder than I was going to have to. I hated it. And thus, I quickly passed from the numbness of denial into my angry phase.

Like any ADD adult person though, I didn't linger long in any of the phases of grieving over my diagnosis. I denied it for about a day or two, projected my anger out on the loving support of my friends and family for about a week, felt hopelessly awkward over the idea of wearing a sparkly pink ribbon for about two more weeks after that, and then I accepted it and moved on. I still didn't want to actually talk to anyone about it, though.

My final breakthrough, however, was when a well-meaning friend outed me on my Facebook page. "*We love you so much and we want you to know how devastated we are and that we're all are here for you and will lift you up in our prayers*!!"

Ack! I panicked. I totally freaked out. Within seconds of my discovery of the post, I was getting all kinds of "OMG" responses to it. In horror, I frantically deleted the post off my wall; then I paced the room like a wet, spitting cat for about an hour. After that, I took a deep breath and logged back on to my Facebook page to let the entire world know. I openly announced to all my friends, acquaintances, family, and people I only knew vaguely through the writing and science fiction communities, what my diagnosis was and what I was about to do.

The response truly humbled me, and like a bolt out of heaven, my apprehensions lifted, and my sense of humor came pouring back. Like the writer I am, I felt free to begin to journal my experiences ~ releasing my anxiety even more. I suddenly wanted to share with everyone what I was going through and that, hard as it might be, was when I vowed I wasn't about to lose my sense of humor over it. It turns out I really needed it.

9
Slipping Off the Sorry Rope

I wish I could say I came to my new-found state of acceptance with dignity and graciousness, but unfortunately, it took a long, long while for me to allow and consent to the good intentions behind each gasp of horror and response of, *"I'm soooo sorry!"*

I began to seriously hate the phrase: "I'm sorry!" Sorry for what? What is…is. I'm dealing with it, and it's okay. I have a stupid lump in my breast, which I'm going to cut out and throw into the furnace, and then I'm getting on with life. I'm too busy not to.

I got as worked up over the reaction of other people as I did the actual diagnosis. I wondered why they couldn't just say something like, *"Grab it and growl, Toots!"* or *"The odds are in your favor, sweetheart!"*

Honestly, the very best thing someone said to me was along the lines of, *"Don't let anyone tell you that you can't pee during chemo. Just stand up and wheel the stupid pole into the stall with you; you'll be totally fine.*" This kind of response, however, was a rarity.

Only gradually did I come to release my irritable angst and realize that they weren't actually sorry for me at all. They were simply trying to reach out with good intentions and sympathize: to give me hope, courage, and strength— all of which I desperately needed to get well (even if I didn't want to admit I needed them).

I don't think I ever really got over being peeved by the "I'm sorry" factor, but I did learn to smile, receive it graciously, and absorb all the good intentions and strength that were meant by it. The weirdness I felt over someone actually wearing pink for me ~ and being so proud to show me ~ took a lot longer, but we can talk about that later.

Like anything in my life, however, there's always something that I can find bafflingly humorous about it all. I can't tell you the number of people who, with all good intentions and absolutely no malice at all, would tell me the most outrageous stories of friends and family and friends of friends who had battled cancer and been just devastated by it. They shared graphic descriptions of dead babies, wasted lives, tortured families, and orphaned children who turned to drugs after mom died in agony. ***Hello! Um...can you see the cancer warrior right in front of you ~ worrying about her own two kids and family?***

I've never quite figured out why people would reach out in this particular way. They really were trying to connect with me just as much as the "*I'm-sorry*" and the "*I'm-praying-so-hard-for-you*" folks, but it would happen over and over again. For every person who assured me they knew survivors of twenty, thirty, or forty years or more, there was someone right there telling me about a girlfriend who had died and left three poor kids under the age of six with a pitiable, grieving, and totally overwhelmed widowed father. And you know what? I would find myself saying that dratted phrase right back to them, *"Oh, my God ~ I'm so, so, sorry!"* You would think, if I hated it so much, that I wouldn't use it ~ right? *Wrong*. Life is so bizarre sometimes.

The best of these morbid outreaches was at my kids' back-to-school event. I was standing with one of my fellow Girl Scout leaders, having the best conversation about scouts and kids, when the husband of one of my other friends interrupted. With honestly good intentions, he just had to tell me that he was *so-oo-oo sorry* and *so-oo-oo devastated* when he heard about my diagnosis. Apparently his co-worker ~ a great big tough, burly, six-foot something, powerhouse of a construction logger-lumber jack ~ had also been diagnosed a few months before, and it had just been horrible for him and his family. The poor guy had gone through surgery after surgery, radiation, chemo ~ you name it. He was just wasting away before everyone's eyes and was now thin, frail, pathetic, and just a walking death corpse itself.

My horrified friend politely tried her best to stop his long, involved, and painfully detailed descriptions of vomiting and the blood and the pain and the wasting, but he just kept on and on, until honestly, I didn't know whether to freak out or cry. (I was only a few days away from my scheduled double mastectomy at this point.) Finally, I just burst out laughing. I really kinda wish I hadn't; it was pretty mean of me. I honestly did my best to hide it behind a feigned choking on my coffee, but all I could do was mutter, "*I'm sooo sorry,*" and excuse myself on some lame pretense that I doubt anyone present believed. Unfortunately, I continued laughing so hard that I turned heads and had to actually step outside the building or risk people thinking I'd completely gone around the bend. To make things worse, when I came back in, my poor girlfriend was still nodding politely ~ a dismayed look on her face ~ totally stuck and patiently still listening to the rest of the gruesome tale.

10
Don't Feed The EOBs

For those who aren't yet aware, an EOB is the "Explanation of Benefits" sent to you via first class mail from the insurance company every time you have a medical test, see a medical doctor, or have any kind of a health-related procedure performed on you or on your behalf. An EOB is not a bill, but it could potentially become a bill; it just depends on the phase of the moon in relation to the tide on the opposite coastline and your astrological sign factored with a formula related to, but not necessarily, Greek numerology.

It outlines the total cost of the procedure, as submitted by your doctor, and how much the insurance company will, or will not, actually pay on your behalf. It's totally based on the insurance company's interpretation of what the claims representative thinks, at the time, is or is not covered by your particular policy. Hopefully, your claim passes across this anonymous claims desk after lunch but before the said claims agent starts stressing out over making his or her kid's music recital after work.

In the United States ~ unless you're in the military ~ when you're diagnosed with cancer, the EOBs start arriving almost on a daily basis and very quickly become a mountain of paperwork. They're supposed to tell you that the claim is under review, but more often than not, they simply freak you out. Fortunately, I have a very überly organized hubby, who could keep it all straight for me ~ most of the time.

After listening to him ranting and muttering to himself in his office downstairs, I came to the conclusion that what EOB should stand for is "Expletives Over Bafflement." Mind you, my husband is an attorney ~ an attorney who has represented our insurance company. Even he couldn't figure out how they arrived at the portion of the bill the policy would, or would not, cover ~ let alone what we'd need to pay out of pocket. I really did feel bad for him. At this point in the treatment, I'd had so many doctor and lab visits that I was automatically handing over my driver's license and insurance card in the grocery store checkout line. I think we were receiving a minimum of two or three EOBs in the mail each week, sometimes more.

The most basic part of this process begins with the co-pay. That's actually simple enough. If the doctor is in-plan, then the co-pay is somewhere around ten dollars. If the doctor is in the group, then the co-pay is twenty dollars. If the doctor is a specialty doctor, or maybe you're going for a well visit, then the co-pay is thirty dollars; unless it's fifty dollars. Regardless, the co-pay is the amount, given up front that you will never see again, and it may or may not be part of the bill submitted. It might be that you won't owe the doctor or laboratory anything after the co-pay is forked over, but, if you want to be seen, then you've got to hand over the cash up front.

The most outrageous co-pay, in my humble and insurance-illiterate experience, was the phone call from the hospital calculating what my portion of my two- to three-day stay in their facility was estimated to be ~ including the fees for the surgery room itself. They called me, a freaked-out cancer patient, three days before I was scheduled for a double mastectomy, to tell me that my part of the bill, due upfront, was $7,000 and that I could not be admitted for the removal of my tumors until it was paid in advance. They did, however, inform me that I was very lucky. Through their processing of my claim, they'd discovered that I'd reached my max payout for the year; so they were only going to charge me $4,000. Would I like to pay via MasterCard, Visa, or American Express?

After the co-pay, however, there's a baffling cryptogram of just how much will be paid ~ toward which doctor, which visit, which test, which procedure, and at which time ~ given the codes provided. I could possibly owe the physician or laboratory nothing, $14.92, $114.29, $0.37, or $4,280. Don't even get me started about the checks mysteriously sent to us and not the doctor. Half the time we couldn't figure out to whom the checks belonged to until the doctor's office actually called and asked for it. Even then we crossed our fingers.

Now, I'm sure there is a perfectly reasonable method that insurance companies follow, and yes, everyone at customer service was incredibly nice every time I called, but if my husband, the lawyer, couldn't figure it out, how the heck does a stay-at-home mom? It's almost like they spin a wheel or throw a dart on a board pasted with random numbers.

At one point, I was informed by one laboratory that even though I'd reached my max payout for the year, that was only for hospital facility use. I hadn't actually reached my max payout for my lab work. *Huh*? Did that mean I still had individually different max payouts for the surgeon, the gynecologist, the reconstruction surgeon, and my oncologist or were all those covered under the umbrella of all said physicians being specialists? How about my primary care physician? Why did his co-pay go up to thirty dollars if he's a group primary and not a specialist? Is that just because I have cancer now?

It honestly wouldn't be so terribly bad, except there's also the very real possibility that the insurance company will make a mistake in its calculations. Errors, it turns out, happen all the time ~ give them their due, the claims clerks are human beings, just like we are ~ but any and all errors are my responsibility to find and that doesn't necessarily mean I can get a refund for the difference. Resubmitting is apparently up to the doctor, or if I don't like it, I can do it myself. That doesn't automatically translate into the reviewed claim resulting in a refund. They might just find another exception in paragraph twelve, sub-section twenty-four-B, page six thousand-twenty-one, and I might just end up owing more.

And I thought battling cancer was hard....

Conquering Mount Ta Ta

11
Nipple Junction

Shortly before my last pre-op before surgery, I
started having these seriously stupid and inane
melodramatic conundrums over the whole
reconstruction issue. Not, mind you, whether I was
going to do reconstruction or not ~ *of course I was*!
The very idea of having pretty, perky little girls again
was simply too good to resist. But all the little details
and options that the plastic surgeon was asking me to
think over gave me a headache. Unfortunately, I had it
locked in my muddled mind that I had to decide on all
the details of my future ideal chest before the
mastectomy ~ which wasn't quite true. As a result, I
found myself seriously OCD over the idea as the
surgery date grew closer. I could only describe it as:
The great nipple conundrum.

As if the stress of having cancer weren't enough,
now I had the anxiety of designing my future best

girlfriends. Nipples…to nip or not to nip: that was the question that totally kept me up at night and nearly gave me an ulcer. Did I want to reconstruct artificial nipples or not? *We should all have these problems, right*? But seriously, it was like building a house and being asked where you want the electrical outlets and what kind of outlets you want ~ *ack!* I mean, size, shape, and filling I could pretty easily handle: less is more. But nipples? I just didn't know!

I knew, without a doubt, that I wanted a smallish size A/B. After years of an annoying two-second lag time while doing flying jumps and kicks, I had totally lost any sentimental attachment to large mammary accessories. The rest I really never thought about considering. I just assumed I would announce my intended bra size, and the plastic surgeon would simply take the lead and give me his best product ~ right? *Oh, how wrong I was*! There was so much more to consider; it gave me migraines.

The whole anatomically precise nipple concept or the smooth braless option; the 3-D tattoo mock up or the works plus; what color ~ *what color? Seriously*? I'm talking about details far more comprehensive than I really want to discuss. There were far too many decisions of a nature that I was just not ready start contemplating. I simply couldn't go there; you know?

And my poor, stoic, no-nonsense hubby: he was just no help at all. I know he had an opinion lurking somewhere in the depths of his male brain. We've been married long enough for me to know he was just itching to say something. However, he was not only uncomfortable expressing it, but he also took the most unexpected, *"don't ask, don't tell"* ultra-conservative approach; refusing to even consider it. When I finally asked him point black to please state his opinion (he is, after all, the only other person on the earth ~ besides the doctors ~ allowed to see and touch the new appliances), he just gave me a horrified look. It was the same expression that crosses his face when I ask if I look fat in a dress: the one that says he's not touchin' that question with a ten-foot pole.

Finally, at a loss, I just chose on my own. Screw it; he had his chance ~ you know? In the end, I had to consider that to reconstruct the nipples would have required yet another surgery, which I didn't want. Also, why the hell, after decades of trying not to "nip out" at the wrong times, was I going to put myself in a position of chronic "nipitis?" It would mean I would never again be able to go braless ~ despite a relatively flat size. Let's get real, people: despite my husband's favorite lamentation (that he's married to an immature fourteen-year-old), twenty-something I ain't. I don't need 'em, and I don't want 'em.

It was the braless concept that finally won me over. At my age, I hadn't been without a padded support bra in nearly thirty years; I simply couldn't resist the idea. The realization freed me about as much as the bra-burning ceremonies performed by those women a generation before me. I grinned from ear to ear and sighed a huge sigh of relief. How did my husband feel? I don't know. He gave me the look of a politician's mask and simply nodded, saying he was happy if I was happy ~ *oh yeah, right.*

I did, however, get a good chuckle and found it extremely ironic that I chose the 3-D nipple tattoo. After going to extreme measures to eradicate the last of my twenty-something tats before my kids grew conscious of them, there I was: deciding on getting the most explicitly graphic set I'd ever had.

So tell me, how am I ever going to answer when my teenagers ask me if I have any tattoos? *"Um…it's anatomical, so it's allowed."* No, that could definitely lead to misunderstandings. *"It's…um…reconstruction; when you get your own done, you can choose it too"* ~ oh, Lord, no. *"Um…because they're mine, and you can't have your own until you're forty-mfflmumble-something too, that's why!"*

Oh, the conversations we're going to have with that one!

12
Ta-Ta to the Ta-Tas!

The doctors made their command very explicit: absolutely no wine or alcohol twenty-four hours before my mastectomy. Honestly, I ask you: isn't that just cruel and unusual punishment? It was the one time in my life I could genuinely say I sincerely needed a drink, and it was forbidden to me. So I did what any sensible woman in my position would do: I threw a party.

Of course, I couldn't have a real party in my home the night before surgery, so I threw a virtual one on the Internet and called it, "Ta-ta to the Ta-tas!" I made it an official event on my Facebook page and then sent out e-invitations to those who were on my e-mail list. I asked everyone I knew ~ wherever they might be at happy hour on that day ~ to raise a glass of their favorite beverage, alcoholic or not, in my honor and toast "Ta-ta to the ta-tas!"

I'll be frank: it was a whim. I was full of nervous anxiety and joking around. I didn't really think anyone would respond with anything more than an eye-roll at my latest odd behavior. However, to my surprise, sixty-seven people ~ from across the Americas and from Australia to Europe and the Middle East ~ posted or e-mailed me back that they had raised their glass for me.

The most popular beverage listed, oddly enough, was root beer, followed by water, but I was pleased as spiked punch to see several good mixers and some Jack Daniels in there as well.

The whole thing touched me considerably. I already knew I wasn't alone going into the mastectomy. My family and close friends had rallied around me, and I felt the warmth of their love and the strength they lent to me, but I also realized I had a whole community of people out there who were also thinking of me and wishing me well. It helped tremendously with the nerves and made me smile from ear to ear.

13

Bungee Jumping
Mastectomy Ravine

Just showing up for the mastectomy was hard. I don't think I slept much the night before, but to be completely truthful, I've blocked much of that experience out ~ or, at the very least, lost it somewhere in a morphine-induced stupor. I remember kissing the kids goodbye and heading to the hospital. I remember arriving at the hospital. But the rest is just bits and pieces which have been linked together by fuzzy memories and by what people laughed about afterward.

The whole experience wasn't exactly what I'd call fun, but I don't think anyone really expected that it would be. I had to wait forever in the hospital's pre-surgery waiting room. They called my name, had me change into the classic hospital gown, and there I lay as my mom and husband and pastor filed in around me. At one point, I remember fretting that I didn't have my red allergy band on, and as the staff double-checked my chart, a nurse very quickly unhooked my IV bag and rushed out with it. When the other nurse inquired what she was doing, the first responded that they were about to intravenously give me an antibiotic that I was allergic to.

All this terrified me, but jumping up and bolting was impossible at that point. I apparently looked so panicked that my hubby grabbed my hand, and the pastor began praying. Fortunately, right about then, the infusion of the good stuff took hold, and all I remember from there on out was lots of pretty lights, rainbows, and little multi-colored pony unicorns dressed in surgical scrubs.

Waking up afterward wasn't nearly as hard as I was expecting. At first, thanks to the morphine, there was less pain and more achiness, but I was shocked at how difficult it was to roll out of bed and go to the bathroom. I could barely move anything from the waist up. Even my arms were weak little noodles and refused to lift or push anything ~ not even tissues. It felt like my left arm, where they had removed the lymph nodes, was sewn down to my side.

Fortunately, I have overdeveloped leg muscles from martial arts, so I figured out fairly quickly how to utilize them to move my uncooperative body. However, once I was upright, a whole new set of challenges presented themselves. My center of gravity was all out of kilter. For years, I'd had all this extra weight pulling on my neck and shoulders, and now it was gone. I felt like a toddler trying to figure out how to balance myself.

I was still pretty out of it that first night back to consciousness, but I do remember that my roommate was a retired nurse. She kept fussing at the night staff that they needed to check me for this or that and mumbling that hospitals just weren't what they used to be. I can't even remember her name, but she was a peach. She was in for a double hernia operation, and she was mobile, so if the night staff didn't answer my call right away, she'd get her walker and go hunt someone down. She even got me a dinner plate after hours and the best cup of contraband coffee in the morning. I remember thinking she was a lot like my grandma who had passed away a few years before.

What astounded me even more, though, was how quickly they threw me out. I was told beforehand that I'd have at least one full night per boob ~ maybe one-and-a-half nights. But apparently, and I have to rely on what others told me afterwards because I don't fully remember, some kind of super bug had evaded my floor and they wanted everybody who could go home released. What I was told later is that I was released because I was doing so well. I was up and walking to the bathroom and eating solid food. Whatever the real reason, I was in the car and on my way home after a day and a half.

The clearest memory of that time was of the wheelchair trip to the car. I think the volunteer was ancient enough to have served in the First World War. He was very nice, but instead of taking me down the smooth, concrete sidewalk, he rolled me down a more direct route via the decorative brick path: one that forced him to zig-zag me back and forth to control the bouncing. Then and there, the drugs abandoned me. As I bumped and rocked from brick to heinous brick, I felt like the slapstick victim of a Saturday night comedy show. Obviously, I must have seriously pissed him off in some former life, and this was his chance to get even for it. I remember my mom running after him and calling for him to stop ~ I'd just had a double mastectomy, so please don't bounce me around ~ but apparently his hearing aide batteries were dead.

No amount of happy juice, however, prepared me for the first unveiling of my bandages in my upstairs bathroom. It had to be done. By that, I mean the bandages had to be changed and the wounds cleaned. But it really would have been nice to have experienced that under the careful guidance of a nurse. Instead, what awaited me in my bathroom mirror were the sad and sagging deflated remnants of former glory days. I'm not talking about the post-nursing kind of droop. I'm talking about the total lack of any kind of cleavage and a sort of concave hole that was covered with wilted, puckering skin. Two long and angry looking lines of stitches stretched from armpit to armpit, with only a little break in the center of my chest. Four clear tubes ~ two on either side ~ drained the most morbidly fascinating fluid out of my chest.

It was like something out of a really bad horror movie or maybe more like a final exam project for a special-effects student. My nipples were gone ~ which was the weirdest part ~ and the rest looked…odd. I just stood and stared at myself in the bathroom mirror. "*Oh my God,*" I thought. "*I've got Frankenboobs!*"

Conquering Mount Ta Ta

14
Cyborg Pass

Nothing ~ I repeat, nothing ~ can ever prepare you for the post-mastectomy experience. Like all those child-rearing books that I poured over when I was a brand new, expectant mother for the very first time, everything everybody tells you will, to some degree, be completely wrong ~ or at least totally useless. I suppose this is because, like every child, everyone wakes up to their new boobless reality just a little differently.

I would love to somehow have an in-depth discussion and give a nod, or at least pay tribute, to the genuine loss of femininity many woman feel ~ which I would never, ever discount ~ but for me at least, the unexpected alteration in my center of gravity was far more disconcerting than the loss of my two aging, womanly power-points. Once the initial adjustment to the pain and the shock of my new Frankenboobs had passed, I began to realize how good those flat-chested men actually have it. What I wasn't prepared for, however, was the cyborg effect.

When so much of the tissue and skin and muscle are removed, there are, of course, repercussions. I had a wonderful pre-op nurse and advocate, who took a whole hour to explain things like: drains, Novocain tubes that deflate to apple cores, support girdles, and tissue expanders. She even had a brilliant little basket of what all the objects looked like and would hand them to me one by one. In the office, everything looked nice, tidy, clinical, and not a problem. However, attached to my sore, bruised, and aching chest, it was a completely different story.

This was the first time in my journey that I completely lost my sense of humor ~at least for a few hours. While being slowly weaned of the blessed morphine, I had some very choice words for my new "sewn-on" appendages. Side note: my Girl Scout Brownies, heck my Cub Scouts, can do prettier stitches than those wires.

There were four long tubes of plastic that had been jammed into my body. These gave a full view of the yellow and red, murky drainage of bodily grossness from the depths of my traumatized chest. These were all attached to ~ and I'm really not kidding here ~ four palm-sized, plastic suction creatures that were heavy and warm and had to be squeezed dry every so often: just like oversized teenage pimples. They were like enormous, mutant deer ticks. I felt hideous, inhuman, and completely incensed over the mutilation of my body. It's very interesting to note that I was not angry over the actual loss of my cleavage; it was the dang plumber's tubing associated with it. I had suddenly turned from a human female into some grotesque caricature ~ and it totally pissed me off.

Physicians used do stuff like this in the Middle Ages. They'd "bleed" their patients and attach leeches and other god-awful creatures to "draw out" the bad humors. Let me tell you, my doctors and caretakers got the bad humors drawn out of me in those first few days. My dearest son referred to my face as having a "puma" look, and my sweet mother, who stayed up for the first seventy-two hours of my return home to care for me 24-7, simply admitted I was a little cantankerous for a while.

I don't know how anyone deals with those stupid drains. It's not like you can simply close your eyes and avert them. They are a constant presence, and since they are a direct pathway into your body, they must be cleaned and cared for like your most pampered pets ~ even if you despise them. I doubt I will ever be able to smell rubbing alcohol again without growling. As my son said, I always smelled like "a shot from the doctor."

There are two ways to secure these blood- and fluid-sucking "ticks" to your body for convenient storage and transport. You can either purchase a Velcro belt (with room for four), or you can just safety-pin them somewhere and let them hang off you. I chose the former option, which, despite making me look like a middle-aged pregnant woman, gave me the best option for tucking the tubes closer to my body and keeping them from popping out at disturbingly odd angles under my shirts: which, by the way, caused some pretty amusing looks on the faces of my visitors as they tried to figure out what was going on under my robe. Someone had advised me beforehand to purchase a few button-down shirts before the surgery, but they had forgotten to mention that I needed shirts at least two sizes bigger to accommodate my new appendages.

The other gross thing no one told me about was the underarm hair. Because of the stitches, I couldn't shave under my arms for the longest time. At one point, I remember grumbling that I was going to braid it with pony beads.

If I had really planned things out better, I think I would have scheduled the surgery the week before Halloween. That way, I could have simply donned a mask and sat on the front porch, completely bare chested, in all my tubed-up glory, and thrown wrapped candy at the horrified neighborhood children. I totally think I would have been a shoe-in for best special effects makeup. I must admit though, it probably wouldn't have been the best way to encourage warm and fuzzy feelings with the other moms on my block.

Don't let them fool you either: the removal of these ticks and tubes is almost as bad as dealing with them 24-7; it hurts like hell. On the brighter side of life, they're only in for a few weeks and the removal is over in seconds. *Lamaze breathing ~ remember that?* Find your focus object, breathe, count to ten, and you'll be just fine. And, as the last one slides from your body, you can grab it, toss it to China (where it was probably made, by a man), and reclaim your humanity once more. Then, like a sixties flower child, you can glory in going about braless for a while.

Conquering Mount Ta Ta

15
Rocky Road

Considering the mastectomy, the first part of
reconstruction was fairly easy for me. In my case, I
didn't qualify for immediate reconstruction, so I went
with the two-stage, delayed reconstruction. After the
initial mastectomy, I had a second surgery,
immediately following, where they implanted two
"tissue expanders." The tissue expanders look like
mini, rectangular heating pads which slide under the
pectoralis muscles under your chest. The idea behind it
is to slowly "pump up" the expanders with saline ~
which will make room for the implants later on. Once
again, I was struck by the idea of rectangular storage
bags making way for round implants ~ *and yes, I found
out that they were, indeed, invented by a man.*
   Once the first set of tubes was removed, they started

filling these skin stretchers ~ excuse me, tissue expanders ~ with massive injections of saline. This process, which lasted a total of five weeks for me, I respectfully named, "the inside-out racking."

In order to reach the "racker" under my chest, the doctor had to locate the self-sealing "opening" of the sack with a magnetic locator, then slip a four-inch, IV-like needle through the muscle and into the bag. The surgeon would then proceed to push an insane amount of saline fluid through the IV until the bag began to "inflate." It's not really as barbaric as it sounds. Well…actually it is, but you really do get used to it. I just kept in mind that I was voluntarily choosing to be racked every Monday for five weeks in order to get a brand new twenty-something's rack. That helped ~ sort of.

Apparently, in order to go down to a B, I had to go back up to a D so the surgeon would have enough skin to work with. I sort of understood that. I guess he figured I might decide at the last minute to be full size again, so he'd need enough to work with ~ just in case. Still, as I slowly and sorely stretched from flat chested back into queen sized, I had more than one moment where I wondered if it was really worth it.

Most women, I'm told, lose almost all sensation in their chest after a double mastectomy. It's the biggest complaint patients have. Some women even say that they can't feel people hugging them anymore. This, fortunately, was not the case with me. I kept well over 90 percent of the feeling in my chest. Unfortunately, this also meant that the racking sessions were that much more painful and difficult to get through. The worst part was the pinch of the needle going through the muscle ~ kind of like a tetanus shot each week ~ and then the burning as the saline went in and filled the racking sacks. This expanded the muscle outward and gave me a rock hard, totally fake chest.

Now, I'm no stranger to pulled or overworked muscles, but it's an entirely different feeling altogether when the expansion is under your boobless chest. Have I mentioned that they can also leak? All of a sudden, I was having flashbacks to my breastfeeding years. The first time, the saline dripped out of the open wound left by the removal of the left tube: at least, I think that's where it came from ~ based on the stain on my shirt. The second and third times, I "leaked" out the injection site. At first, I panicked and thought something was terribly wrong, but apparently, it happens all the time and no one at the plastic surgeon's office seemed overly concerned. It would have been nice if I'd been warned ahead of time, but after a while, I became an old pro and simply changed my shirts without thinking twice about it.

What I never did get quite used to were the spasms. During this procedure, the muscles of the chest will "spasm" as they adjust to the pressure of the saline-filled pouches against them. Have you ever seen those body builders at the gym who make their pecs jiggle up and down because they think women will find it sexy? (*Not!*) Well, it's the same sort of thing. With the skin stretchers though, the spasms and wiggling are totally random and you can't control them. I called it *the boobie-hoochie-coochie.*

At first, it's not really noticeable to the outside world, but because the skin has to be stretched a little bigger than the implant, as I grew larger and larger, so did my boobie dance. Sweatshirts. I definitely recommend hubby-sized sweatshirts. The doctor also suggested Valium, but that worked more to relieve the stress of my children bickering rather than the ripples and twinges in my chest. It eventually settled down, but then I figured out how to control the chest muscles up and down and side to side on my own ~ which totally grossed out my kids. It brought out the worst of my impish humor, and quite possibly, scarred both of them for life ~ but it was fun.

The drunken knocker dance, however, wasn't the end of the story. The feeling of the liquid sliding through the rectangular pouches and the popping of the edges of the bags nipping outward in weird directions ~ it all felt like I was being groped from the inside out. It was seriously weird and made sleeping a completely new and decidedly odd experience.

After the tubes came out, I was desperate to get off the foam wedge and sleep on my side again. What I didn't realize was that those stupid skin stretchers are really heavy and as hard as rocks. Not only did the muscles over them do that random, spasmodic, and involuntary disco, but the sacks themselves were uncomfortable when I put any kind of pressure on them by rolling over. With all of this combined, it basically prevented me from sleeping for a while.

In the end, I figured out a way to take two standard-sized pillows and lay them on either side of me. I would tuck the side of the pillow in-between the fake mounds, and it would relieve just enough pressure to be relatively comfortable. I ended up naming them Hans and Franz ~ because they were there to "prop" me up.

Conquering Mount Ta Ta

16

Snakeskin

Ecdysis is the fancy, scientific, name for the shedding of snakeskin. It's also called sloughing or molting and absolutely no one warned me that this is exactly what happens around the mastectomy incisions. I mean, I was doing just fine until I started peeling like a reptile and dropping huge flakes of grey, slightly moist dead skin everywhere. I'm not quite sure if it was really just the skin over the incision, the stretching skin over the expanders, the scabs drying out and taking the stretching skin with them, or some kind of weird mixture of skin and the glue used nowadays to close the incision. Regardless, it's *gross*, but it's also kind of fascinating ~ in a morbid kind of way.

By four weeks out, I was actually feeling pretty well. I was slowly getting back into the routine of being a mom, but I was not quite ready for prime time yet. I would have these huge bursts of energy, then I'd come crashing down and totally wipe out, completely unconscious, in deep sleep on the sofa ~ drooling. If you have nice children like I do, they'll take a picture of it and post it on Facebook.

All the "new" activity pinched a lot, but I was growing accustomed to the chronic, never-ending soreness and achiness. I chalked up the burning and itching (like an ant infestation) to just the normal healing of a really big wound or maybe because I'd overdone it a little and pulled the incision too hard. I really did try to listen to my body while recovering, but I also pushed myself ~ until my chest started molting.

At first, I thought it was simply the scabs drying out or maybe the skin was being stretched a little too fast. It was about the right time for it, and I was glad. I was ready to move past the last remaining symbols of the cyborg phase and concentrate on reconstruction. It soon became evident, however, that this was not your normal incision healing. There were just a few flakes at first ~ like boob dandruff ~ then big, long strips…like snakeskin. It was a perversely captivating phenomenon but not exactly something you want to share with others ~ *you know*?

After a day or two, I started wearing a sports bra again: not for support, but to catch the soft chunks of grey, dead skin and scabs that would fall off at inconvenient times. I think my son was unfairly maligned at one point for picking his nose and leaving it on the couch, but I was too wimpy to admit it was probably something that accidentally dropped off one of my boobs. Clorox wipes became my new best friend.

Showering in the mornings became a ghastly obsession with me. I'd loofa as much as I could tolerate, pull as much of the dead skin wads off as I could, and then moisturize the heck out of the remaining tendrils ~ mocking me like the remnants of a bad, peeling sunburn. By nightfall, those little remnants would be long strands again, and I'd start all over with the loofa and the moisturizer.

I was assured by other mastectomy survivors that this was a perfectly normal occurrence, but if it was so perfectly normal, why didn't anyone tell me about it? I suppose it's a little like childbirth and the new mother. Everyone focuses on the joy of the baby being delivered, but no one ever mentions the slime, the blood, and the gunk the baby actually arrives in. After a while, mammary skin-shedding maintenance simply became part of my wound management, but I was very glad to see this particular phase come to an end.

Conquering Mount Ta Ta

17
Blue Skies

"BEST NEWS EVER!!!!"

This is what I wrote on my CaringBridge.com journal page on Friday, October 12th. It was the first day of the rest of my life.

I already knew that by opting for the big kahuna, the double mastectomy, I wouldn't need radiation, but chemotherapy infusions still hadn't been ruled out. I knew my tumors were small, I knew the 3-D mammogram had caught my cancer early, I knew they had gotten everything out, I knew they took the left lymph, but I didn't know my risks for getting cancer again. My oncologist really didn't help. He kept changing his mind back and forth with my surgeon: *"Well...she's young...but then again...on the other hand...."* Finally, the decision was made to send my tumor out to be gene evaluated ~ just to make sure.

This is the most brilliant thing about cancer therapy nowadays. Just a few years before me, there would have been no question about chemotherapy. It was a one-size-fits-all approach. Now, however, cancer treatment is very specialized. They can map the actual genes that make up a tumor and find the specific medicine and treatment options that work the best for it. In my humble opinion, this is the greatest marvel to develop, like a blessed gift, from all the other cancer warriors before me. It was simply amazing to me that, by testing for something like sixteen specific genes, they can pretty much tell what kind of specially designed treatment is going to work the best.

I was eager for my follow-up with the oncologist that afternoon, but I was also dreading it. The tumors had been sent to California and I kind of felt like I was awaiting the results of a mid-life college entrance test. It seemed like one test was going to determine my whole future.

My rating came back at fourteen out of one hundred, and for the first time in my life, I was incredibly happy to get such a low score on a test. Better yet, they determined that my recurrence score was only nine percent (Nine is my lucky number). That meant that there would be no infusions ~ just Tamoxifen for five to ten years. It would not be the terrifying IV drip I was so scared of. My results were positioned right on the upward corner of the V on the bar graph: where chemotherapy infusions combined with Tamoxifen would not necessarily be more helpful versus

Tamoxifen alone. If I hadn't had the 3-D mammogram when I did, it might have been a completely different story.

I felt as if I could breathe again. *I was going to keep my hair*! (Well, most of it. It still turned grey overnight and came out in handfuls, but few noticed.)

I didn't know whether to laugh, cry, giggle, or burst into tears. It was over. Well, not really, but it felt like it was over. I immediately went out and bought nine lottery tickets, but I guess I used up all my luck fighting cancer. Still, I didn't care; I had made it. Now all I had to do was get used to the Tamoxifen and wait for reconstruction at the end of the year.

I had done it! I had won!

Conquering Mount Ta Ta

18
Unexpected Detours

Alright, so maybe I was a little ahead of myself in declaring victory. I guess my real problem was that my short-term goals had been a little short sighted. What had mattered most to me going into this was to cut the cancer out and pray that I didn't have to have radiation and chemo infusions. When those two desires came to fruition, I thought I was done, and it was easy sailing ~ even though I would still have to take cancer medications in pill form. Unfortunately, I couldn't have been more wrong.

With every life-threatening illness, there are always setbacks, and my particular challenge was to accept them with slightly better grace than a petulant three year old that wasn't getting her way. I seriously misjudged how achy and sore I'd be after three months of skin stretchers under my chest, but I underestimated even more how tough the Tamoxifen was going to be.

Unbeknownst to me, all the stress ~ and, I admit it, all the extra red wine ~ associated with my diagnosis and treatment had really done a number on my stomach. It was irritated and in full, outright rebellion by the time of my little victory lap and the consumption of my first T-pill (T for Tamoxifen). Although I took it with a full glass of water, by the twelve-hour mark, I was writhing in pain. We're talking pain that I haven't experienced since I was nine months pregnant with my son and suffering acute appendicitis.

My oncologist assured me it couldn't be the Tamoxifen. In all his years, he'd never seen gastritis and gastroparesis develop so quickly. Those were symptoms that rarely occurred, and then, if they did, they only occurred after years of exposure. The doctors were baffled, but they eventually decided that I had simply picked up a bug at my primary doctor's office ~ I'd just been to see him for a case bronchitis.

Unfortunately, by the second week of not being able to eat solid food, the idea of a gastritis bug had to be put aside. I'd lost eleven pounds by this point ~ which, honestly, wasn't entirely a bad thing ~ but I couldn't go another week on liquids and chicken broth alone. I kept trying to insist that wine was a liquid, but neither my doctors nor my stomach would tolerate the idea.

The gastroenterologist who took over at this point was a life saver. He took me off of Tamoxifen and put me on a course of other medicines to calm my rebellious gut down. Then he began an investigation

into whether I had an ulcer or if I'd picked up Giardia
on a scout trip somewhere. Like a miracle, after only a
few days, I was able to start back on crackers, then
noodles, then mushy vegetables and finally real food
again. An endoscope revealed ten areas of my stomach
and small intestine which were irritated and inflamed ~
but there were no actual ulcers ~ as well as a stomach
polyp and a hiatal hernia. There was, however, still no
real idea of what was actually going on. Still looking
for the right clue that would lead to the root of the
problem, he ordered more tests.

At this point in my treatment, you'd think nothing
would faze me, right? I mean, I'd dealt with the
diagnosis of cancer, handled all the poking and
prodding and testing, and survived the mastectomy and
everything associated with it ~ *what could possibly
bother me about more lab tests*?

I knew I was in trouble when I arrived at the lab, and
the technician took me over to a private corner: *uh-oh*.
She then preceded to hand me three prescription pill
containers with fluid inside and something that looked
suspiciously like my children's old potty-training seat:
you know ~ the kind that fits over the toilet but has a
little bowl under it to keep things from dropping into
the water itself. She then explained that I needed to
take everything home, wait for my bowels to start
moving, and gather a good size sample in the collection
pan. *Okay*….

She also gave me very specific directions about
placing just enough "*specimen*" in each tube to bring
the fluid up to a specific line: no more, and no less. I

also had to be very precise about marking each cylinder with the exact time and date the "*sample*" was added. Then I was to put the tubes in a biohazard bag and place them in my refrigerator until I could drive them back to the lab ~ *eww*.

Alright ~ reality check here: I'm a mom of two kids, I'm a black belt in martial arts, and I'm a cancer warrior. I can handle taking specimens of my own poop, right? ***Wrong***.

I'm not entirely sure what I expected. I knew that at least two or three of the tests my doctor ordered required fecal samples, but I really thought they'd give me a gown, tell me to bend over, and that would be the end of my participation in the matter; no pun intended. I mean, that's the way they do it at the vet's office: *just lift the tail, and….*

I hate to admit it, but I avoided going home. I tossed the bulky specimen shield in the back of the van and blocked it out of my mind. I ran more errands on the way home from that lab than I had in the entire time since I'd come home from my mastectomy. Unfortunately for me, by about the fifth or sixth errand, my morning coffee kicked in, and there was no denying I'd have to go home and at least try to face the plastic potty. This was one aspect of fighting cancer that I was just not prepared for.

Fortunately for me, it was one of those rare moments in time when the house was completely empty. The kids were at school, hubby was at work, and my parents had gone out to run their own errands. Relieved beyond measure to find myself alone, I quickly climbed the stairs and secreted myself away in the master bathroom. Now, I've done plenty of camping with the scouts, and I've been faced with some fairly challenging situations in which to get daily personal business done, but this was up there among the most uncomfortable. I can honestly say that I have a new-found respect for toddlers who just can't stand to sit on a practice potty; *it's creepy*.

Once things were accomplished, however, the, um, "*sample*," had to get from the pan to the specimen containers ~ without spilling any of the liquid already inside those containers. It's not like I would get a second shot at this either. I had exactly one tube per test requested. If I screwed up, I'd have to go back to the lab and start over. However, this particular part of the puzzle hadn't been explained by the technician. I got the concept: take things from point A to point B…but with what? *Gross*.

A quick investigation of the kitchen and garage for single-use plastic or paper supplies yielded nothing. My mother, God bless her, had utilized the time I was bedridden to clean out my entire kitchen and storage areas, so there was absolutely nothing disposable left in the house ~ not even leftover party napkins. In the end, I snatched one of the dog poop bags from my dog's leash, held my nose, winced, made several contorted faces my kids would have been proud of, and completed the task with as much dignity as I could muster ~ which wasn't much. I mean, *don't they put people into mental institutions for playing with stuff like this?*

Once the collection tubes were sealed and placed inside the bio-hazard bags, I simply couldn't stand the idea of placing them inside my refrigerator. I mean, *really*? That goes against every ingrained "momism" there is. In the end, I climbed back in the van and drove all the way back to the lab, waited about an hour for another technician, and then dropped the whole thing off in the same day. Breathing a huge sigh of relief, I drove straight home. When my mother asked where I'd been all day, I answered, *"Playing with poop."*

19
Survival Skills

So, when exactly are you a cancer survivor? I was really surprised by all the different answers I got to this question. Most people agree that you're a survivor once you're declared cancer free ~ but just when that is, is a source of some fairly heated and emotional debate.

There are those who believe that you are a survivor the minute the cancer is cut out and the lab decides that the margins are good and clear; others feel this isn't really so because the first two years are a critical benchmark. This two-year period is the highest window for a missing cell to start a new tumor. For this reason, many people insist that you're only really in remission for the first two years and possibly even the five to ten years you're on Tamoxifen. Then there's a group who point out that your chances of the cancer coming back is also a lot higher ten to fifteen years down the road. The more I researched, the more I began to wonder if anyone was actually a "survivor."

It really is amazing how humans, especially women, can bicker over the silliest of details. I don't suppose it really matters when you choose to call yourself a survivor, but the thought of it seemed to perpetually bug me. I was sore, I was tired, and I really wasn't anywhere near ready to call my fight to the top of Mount Ta-Ta over quite yet. Maybe I could think of myself as getting there, but I hadn't really reached the end of my journey.

In the end, I decided it was a personal choice. What you call yourself ~ whether "*in remission*" or a "*survivor*" ~ is more based on how you feel inside. Is the battle really over, or are you still fighting?

Personally, I was still fighting. My stomach was being eaten raw from the inside out, and I was, I admit it, an emotional basket case. So I chose the remission route. On each month's anniversary of my surgery, I counted: "*One month's remission...two months' remission...three months' remission....*" By month three, I was feeling a lot more like my old, pre-cancer self. Best of all, it marked the end of the horrid tissue expanders and reconstruction!

20
Holiday Rock Slides

By the end of November, I was celebrating my second month of remission. The day the holiday carols started playing on the radio, I skipped into an overdrive of excitement and pulled out all the previously bought presents I had to wrap. As I sat there on the family room floor ~ covered with tape and paper and singing along with the music until the dog literally couldn't take it anymore ~ everything suddenly came crashing down and hit me like a ton of bricks. The reason I had so many presents to wrap was because I had pre-bought many of the things on the kids' anticipated wish list. I had pre-bought, because I hadn't known if I'd be well enough to shop or not before Christmas.

At the most thankful and joyous time of my life, I suddenly became completely and overwhelmingly depressed. I've had my share of blue moods before, but

I've never had something that just clung to me like a wet blanket and refused to go away for days on end. It was almost terrifying. I had to force myself to move, to get dressed, or to even walk the dog. It wasn't like me at all, and when both kids suddenly got sick at the same time, I felt like the whole world was coming to a hopeless end.

About this time, one of the younger siblings of a player on my son's hockey team asked if I was really my son's mom or if I was his stepmom. I had missed so many practices and games since my surgery that she wouldn't believe I was who I said I was ~ even when my daughter stepped in and assured her that I was really their mother. I didn't just cry; I wept. I curled into a fetal position. I stayed in my pajamas and even (*gasp*) ignored the Internet and all social media. I drank way too much red wine and consumed most of the kids' leftover Halloween candy. I gained over ten pounds. I am, I have always admitted it, a self-proclaimed drama queen, but this period of my life was unequivocally ridiculous in its spectacle.

The anxiety was the most debilitating. I would wake up at two or three in the morning gasping for air; my heart would be pounding with some unknown fear. I had vivid, brutally terrifying and nasty nightmares. It was as if all the stress and all the trauma of my cancer diagnosis had suddenly revealed itself. It didn't make sense. This was the time that I should have been able to breathe. This was the time to celebrate that the scary part was over, and even though I still had long years of medicine ahead of me, the hard part was over ~ *wasn't it*? I can't explain it, except, perhaps this was the moment that it either dawned on me for the first time exactly how scared I really was, or maybe it was the first moment I allowed myself to be really afraid.

Finally, I sought the help of my primary physician, who assured me that I was having a perfectly normal reaction. He called it something akin to a post-traumatic cancer syndrome. No, of course that isn't a real medical diagnosis, but the idea is the same. All my energies had been focused on battling cancer. I had geared up for the fight and faced it head on, and then suddenly everything stopped and I was supposed to go back to normal: as if I'd never faced this ugly monster and amputated part of my body to destroy it. What I was feeling was normal, but I still had to deal with it.

It took about ten days ~ and some really good prescription medicines ~ for the clouds to finally part. Even then, the anxiety would still propel me out of bed at three o'clock in the morning faster than a hot flash on a snowy night. It seemed absurd to me that I was being so morose now ~ when things were actually looking bright. This was the point I had been waiting for; this was the time to celebrate ~ but I couldn't bring myself to do it.

All the doctors were incredibly pleased with me, yet I couldn't be pleased with myself. Then, like the click of an old-fashioned light switch, one day I woke up and it was gone. I have absolutely no explanation for it other than that it happened. Christmas came and went, and I was happy again, but there was still an odd fatigue lurking just outside my conscious thoughts which wasn't there before and that I couldn't quite shake away.

L.G. Ransom

21
Repelling Down
Reconstruction Slope

Boobs! *Glorious boobs*! No more skin stretchers that slip, ache, and poke at weird angles! That was the one thought that got me through the last few weeks with the tissue expanders. Although my son thought it was hysterical that I'd learned how to bob them up and down independently on command, I was sick of the rock-hard, painful devices. Reconstruction was going to be the best Christmas present ever!

About a week before the surgery, I saw both the mastectomy surgeon and the plastic surgeon, and both seemed very pleased with me. The tissue expander on the left side had slipped and dropped down my chest, but apparently that was a non-issue ~ which was a relief. Apparently slipping out of place happens a lot (*That would have been good to know going in…*). It looked weird and was really uncomfortable, but neither doctor seemed overly concerned. The first surgeon dismissed me for six months ~ *yea! One less fifty-dollar co-pay to worry about*! ~ and she left me to the care of my primary doctor and my plastic surgeon.

My reconstruction date was set for December 28th, which would not only work out great for juggling the kids, but it was also three days before the end of the year ~ and three days before our maximum insurance payout for 2012 ended (*it's the little things in life*). For the first surgery, the hospital usage fee alone was around $4,000, so sliding in before January was huge.

I was, however, very disappointed to learn that I wouldn't be able to go down any smaller than a size C. Apparently, you can only reduce a chest so many sizes before the procedure doesn't work right ~ but why on earth that's so completely eludes me. I mean, in September they had taken everything off, so technically I was starting at ground zero, right? I had been so looking forward to a flat-chested size A or a size B that the concept of a size C really bummed me out for a while. It was, however, much smaller than what I started with, so I finally resigned myself to the fact that you can't always get everything you want.

The other not-so-fabulous news ~ that came out about the same time ~ was of a new study that suggested women with my type of breast cancer should possibly take Tamoxifen for ten years instead of five. I'm still honestly not sure how I feel about this.

Tamoxifen and I really don't like each other very much. Between the stomach issues it causes me, the joint pain, the confusion, the fatigue, the sweats and hot flashes ~ I just don't like it. For me, being on Tamoxifen is like having a chronic case of the flu that never, ever goes away. But, again, it's a pick-your-poison kind of thing.

I've told myself over and over that little white pills are much better than the drip ~ even if they were eating my stomach from the inside out. At this point though, I was actually doing much better in that department. I was on three different medicines that would, hopefully, calm everything down, and ~ best news of all ~ I got to stop the Tamoxifen briefly until after reconstruction. So I was temporarily living large and eating spicy Indian food again!

Conquering Mount Ta Ta

22
One Last Climb

There's always one final push to reach the top of any mountain. By that point, you're usually tired, sore, bruised, and wondering if it's really worth it. This was about how I felt the week before my reconstruction surgery. Consciously, I knew this was a good thing. I really wanted the expanders out, and everyone promised me I'd be so much happier once the implants were in. It was simply the idea of facing another surgery. The IV, the anesthesia, the pain killers ~ *ugh*. I had climbed this mountain for so long that the idea of scaling just one more precipice made me want to rethink everything. I mean, just getting to the base camp is a pretty good achievement. Not everyone has to go all the way up to the oxygen deprived top ~ *right*?

I was more than ready to get rid of the tissue

expanders. The expander on the left (where they took my lymph nodes) had slipped out of place and had a tenancy to drop down and slide outward: toward my arm. It wasn't a huge deal, but I found myself having to closely watch the expressions of the people I encountered. Every once in a while, they'd slow down their words and get a curious look on their faces (especially the guys), which would be my cue to excuse myself, reach under my shirt, and hoist the offending artificial boob out from under my armpit and back to a forward-pointing direction again.

The last few days seemed to drag by and then speed up with holiday craziness all at the same time. As I prepared for what I hoped would be my last surgery (not), once again I found myself banned by the doctors from any and all alcohol the night before. When and where they decided on this rule leaves me shaking my head. Seriously, does it really matter all that much? In the end, I cheated. I had a teeny tiny little shot glass of red wine in the early afternoon ~ all the while reveling in my blasphemous rebellion.

The pre-dawn arrival at the hospital on December 28th was way too early for me to be out and about without the benefit of coffee. The weather was cold and wet and ominous: not helping my nerves at all. Everything about check-in was exactly as it had been before, and I could feel my heart thudding in my chest. When they took me back and handed me the hospital gown, I desperately wanted to go home and call the whole thing off. However, I knew I was stuck. The tissue expanders ~ like it or not ~ had to come out. As long as I was going under anesthesia, I might as well get it over with.

From there, though, despite my blood pressure and my pulse skyrocketing on the monitors, things seemed to go a lot more smoothly than the first time. The very first thing they asked me about was my allergy wrist band ~ which inspired far more confidence in me than with the mastectomy. The new prep team seemed to know what they were doing, and they talked me through each step with a good mixture of caring and confidence that I was in good hands. *Oh, how I wish I'd had that team the first time around*! Even when they couldn't get the IV line into my poor veins, I didn't have nearly as much nervous anxiety over being put to sleep as I had experienced only three months earlier ~ but I was still scared. I remember being wheeled out into the hall and through some doors, and I remember thinking this was more than I remembered the last time. Then, the next thing I knew, they were telling me it was time to go home.

The doctors gave me some pretty good juice when they released me from the hospital that day. I remember waking up ~ or semi-waking up ~ and I remember being loaded into the car, but I have no memory if I walked out or was wheeled out. My mother assures me that I was taken out to the curb in a wheelchair and then proceeded to moan dramatically every time my poor husband turned a corner with the car. My only legitimate memories, however, are: simultaneously being grateful I'd had the foresight to set up the foam wedge and pillows on my bed, complaining to my mother that my bikini underwear had way too much fabric to be considered a bikini, and some murky derogatory remark about my butt fat and being middle aged ~ before falling dead asleep until the next morning.

During this time, I also remember that at least two of my girlfriends called to check on me, but I had absolutely no idea what I said (*The sad thing is that both of them just chuckle and refuse to tell me*).

The next morning I was writhing in over-the-top, dramatic pain. I was completely incensed that everyone had told me reconstruction was an easier surgery and totally bemoaning my poor fate. For two days, I was very vocal about crying foul, but I don't think anyone in the house paid much attention to me. My chest hurt like hell, and I was terrified to see what cyborg nightmare awaited me under the bandages this time.

To my surprise, everything was fairly neat and tidy. I had a few stitches where they had done some liposuction and sculpting, but everything looked like I had real boobs again; minus the nipples of course. It was actually a totally unexpected feeling. I sort of just stared at them blankly and wondered when I was going to spot the part that was going to gross me out ~ but nothing did.

After that initial reaction, I got greedy. On closer examination, the skin was all pitted on the bottom, and things weren't exactly perfectly round. I had deep, monstrous dark purple bruises everywhere ~ which was why I was so sore ~ and my chest certainly wasn't the perfect ideal I had imagined in the beginning. Feeling a bit like an ungrateful child who got a generic tablet instead of the latest and greatest *i-fruit* version, I cleaned myself up, put my surgical corset back on, and stomped back to bed.

By day three, though, I was willing to admit that the second surgery was, indeed, easier than the first. The recovery was definitely quicker, and the pain seemed to not be quite as overwhelming. However, the doctors are right when they say it takes about four weeks; there's no speeding up the healing process. Also, by the end of the first week, I was very happy with my new chest. If I'd had my druthers, I would still have gone another size smaller, but I certainly couldn't complain about the results ~ they were very pretty. The initial dimpling smoothed out as the swelling went down, and they rounded out nicely.

My only complaint, if it's really a complaint at all, was that they felt like cold gel packs permanently attached to my chest. Now I'm the first to admit that- that's not exactly a bad thing during a Tamoxifen induced heat wave, but it definitely took some getting used to and I would have appreciated a heads up about it beforehand. The pros, however, definitely outweighed the cons, and by week four I was feeling pretty good about the whole thing.

Until that point, I hadn't really thought I'd missed having breasts. I was content that the cancer was out and fairly ambivalent about installing new editions, but I have to admit that I was extremely pleased with the end results. I had regained a kind of femininity that I hadn't thought I'd lost.

I had been content with the ravages of children and middle age. I had been accepting of the mutilation of the mastectomy and put on a brave face through the annoyance and un-comfortableness of reconstruction, but now I had something beautiful to show for it. It was a little like regaining a sparkle of youth. The looming fiftieth birthday (still a precious few years away) suddenly didn't seem like such a massive hurdle. It was a very curious experience. Now, if I could just figure out a way to achieve the same results with my chin and buttocks....and my thighs and my...

23
Views From the
Summit of Mt Ta-Ta

"You have to understand," my doctor told me with a serious, yet pleased look, "you're a mammogram success story."

A mammogram success story. That was a very peculiar concept to process. Mine was the outcome that every woman wants when she's diagnosed with breast cancer. I was the statistic that everyone involved in the war against breast cancer is fighting very hard to achieve. Yes, I was ecstatic, but that didn't stop an odd, pesky guilty feeling from welling up in my chest.

I couldn't shake the survivor's guilt. Just knowing that there were many women who don't get to declare victory against cancer took away almost every ounce of joy in my own survival. When my cancer buddy, my mom's sister, passed away shortly after her last round of radiation, I went into a deep depression. How I survived and she didn't, completely baffled and terrified me. We had been fighting cancer together and, in an instant, I was still here and she was gone.

In a nutshell, I felt guilty that I got the chance to live when so many women didn't. I lived because they didn't ~ that's an even more unsettling thought. Their battles paved the way for the 3-D mammogram that found my cancer early, that helped the surgeons understand and perfect the mastectomy, and that helped develop the genetic testing that determined I'd be just fine with only medicine and not infusions. There's a huge responsibility in that. I felt an enormous need to walk a three-day marathon, start a breast cancer ministry at church, or write a book. *One out of three is pretty good, right?*

I have a very good friend who absolutely will not get a mammogram, because it's painful. I have another friend who staunchly does not believe breast cancer even exists at all. I can respect both women for their opinions, but I also know what I experienced ~ and am still experiencing ~ for myself. I now feel like I have a responsibility to all those who came before me and who pioneered the studies that I benefited from to share with all those who will come after. I know without a shadow of a doubt that if I had waited another six months to have my mammogram ~ if I had not had the 3-D mammogram ~ I would be concluding this book on a completely different note. My battle is now pretty much over, but the war against breast cancer is not.

It's not easy for me to throw my shoulders back and say, "*I'm a mammogram success story.*" It's not easy to hear that I'm some sort of glorious culmination of all the women who fought and struggled before me ~ who endured so I didn't have to. But I can say, "*thank you.*" Thank you for all you gave, thank you to all who researched, thank you to everyone who never gave in. Because you never gave up, neither did I...and now I can pass it on.

There's nothing funny about cancer, though humor is awfully good medicine. I can't say I've always been able to maintain my sense of humor at every single twist and turn of my journey, but I sure as hell tried.

Breast cancer is completely scary and utterly life changing. Attitude, however, is everything. It will determine whether you crawl into the fetal position and give up or charge, head first and eyes forward, toward the summit.

My mother often says I dodged a bullet, but I disagree. I took the hit, dug it out, had them stitch me back up, and then proudly showed off my scars like a little kid.

In a way, I kind of feel that I had it easy: not that a double mastectomy is anything to sneeze at. What I mean by that statement is that I conquered my mountain early in the game. I've always been one to rush ahead like that ~ ask anyone who knows me. But this time I got lucky. I got the right diagnosis at the perfect time and became the outcome that every cancer warrior ahead of me fought to achieve ~ *I lived.*

For now though, my battle is pretty much over. As I write this last chapter, I'm marking the first year of my initial diagnoses. I still have the long, five-to-ten-year climb down from the summit I'm calling " *Tamoxifen Trail,* " and I've also capitulated to my neurotic vanity and will schedule the much moaned over nipple reconstruction surgery in the next few months. But the worst, I hope, is now behind me.

I suppose I won't be officially able to say I'm done with cancer until December of 2022 ~ when I take my last Tamoxifen pill ~ but what a New Year celebration that will be! Maybe in ten years, I'll be able to update this and tell you what happens. But for now, I'm on top of the world ~ with beautiful views all around me.

L.G. Ransom

Conquering Mount Ta Ta

About the Author:

L.G. Ransom was born in Miami, Florida but grew up living in various countries around the world.

She's a black belt in Tae Kwon Do, a photographer, an artist, a scout leader, a breast cancer survivor, and lives in the suburbs of Washington DC with her husband, two incredible children, and very spoiled Cavalier King Charles Spaniel.

<u>She says about the subject of breast cancer:</u>

I have a magnet on my refrigerator that states: "Take time to laugh, it's the magic of the soul." I'm not saying dealing with cancer is easy; it's not. But life goes on and beautiful moments still happen. If you allow cancer to destroy the good things in your life, then it wins, and you lose. Living with cancer can be neurotically fast and furious, and if you don't stop and enjoy the good stuff going on all around you, you'll never get those precious minutes back again. However, regardless of any outcome, if you chose to live every beautiful twinkling moment to the fullest, to love, to laugh, and to enjoy life around you, you not only open your heart to that experience, but you become a shining beacon of hope to others around you.

For more information about her books, visit LGRansom.com

Some events and stories in Conquering Mt TaTa were edited and/or combined with others. All are true.

www.ingramcontent.com/pod-product-compliance
Lightning Source LLC
Chambersburg PA
CBHW070538290526
45790CB00002B/553